Doing keto! Keep it simple stupid & lose weight with no exercise.

Loose almost 10 lbs in the first week like I did!

Emma Hector, mother of 6

ISBN:1721902597
ISBN-13: **978-1721902590**

DEDICATION

I dedicate this book to God, Jehovah, creator of heaven and earth for he created us all and without Him nothing would be made. He created our bodies so magnificently and I am blessed to have finally found some of His wisdom in finding the simple, easy and yet most effective way to drop fat weight from of our bodies!

CONTENTS

ACKNOWLEDGMENTS

I would like to acknowledge God first and foremost for blessing me with a beautiful family of six children and a loving husband.   I am so grateful to Him and I am the happiest I can be in my body which is now in great shape without having to work at it physically. The bible is so spot on when God says exercise profits you little!

1 HOW I STARTED AND WHAT DID I WEIGH

I was at the point of discouragement as all the scales said each week was the same figure and sometimes going up a pound or two. On Tuesday 12th March 2018 I weighed 180.0 lbs. The following Tuesday I weighed 182.5 lbs. I weigh myself every Tuesday morning as I get up and before dressing. I would recommend you find a day each week to do the same as this will help and serve as motivation during this lifestyle change!

I found and researched some information on the paleo diet as someone at the bank told me they had started and lost 10 lbs. quickly. It wasn't until I you tubed it that I stumbled upon this new concept that I had never heard or come across before, the "ketogenic diet'. I started to listen and as I read on I could clearly see what success people were having and how effortlessly it was to make this a lifestyle change because the foods that you can eat fill you up and are extremely tasty. I mean who doesn't like bacon and eggs for example?

I began doing keto on Monday March 26th, 2018. My weight the next day dropped to $180.1 lbs. (as I always honor weighing myself every Tuesday morning by habit). I recorded and journaled everything I put into my mouth including beverages so that I could really see if this thing would work. I was excited and couldn't wait to come on board as I know you are! I lost 35.6 lbs. in 3 months by doing this. Be inspired!

2 WHAT FOODS YOU CAN EAT

What I did first was research you tube and learnt a lot about keto / low carb diet. I printed off a spreadsheet which details all what you can and can't eat and other crucial information, each food's carbohydrate count. You want to keep your daily carbohydrate number at 20g or lower for the day and how you log or keep track of this is log your food in an app and weigh all your food. It will pay off and you can stop weighing food when you get accustomed to portion sizes and amounts that make you full up. You just don't want to go over that 20g carbohydrates a day and I stuck to 'total carbs', not net. You'll learn that most ketoer's stick to 20g of net carbs which means that their total carbs maybe for example 50g but then they subtract the fiber content in g to arrive at the 20g NET carbs. This is a way but in my opinion it's not the strongest, so to speak "prescription' way of doing this.

You can eat most vegetables, all the meats, all the cheeses, eggs, real butter, heavy whipping cream but only 2 tablespoons maximum per day, pork rinds, ham and deli meats. You do not have to avoid fats in the meat, in fact they are good for you to eat and help you to stay full and happy until the next meal!

- This diet will provide your body with the nutrition it needs
- It will get rid of the nutritionally 'empty carbohydrates that it does not need which is maintaining your higher weight by a process of keeping your insulin high (you want insulin low to lose weight to) Sugar makes insulin high.
- Can't stress this enough, for EFFECTIVE weight loss like I had, keep your carbohydrate consumption TOTAL at or below 20g

per day. You can trace this by plugging in all what you eat and weigh into the 'Loose it' app and play around with it, to see what your total carbs would be if you ate this or that for your meals and snacks for the entire day. This way you are sure of keeping to that goal.

- If the food is packaged, check the label for the carbohydrate count; 2g or less for meat and diary and 5g or less for vegetables

It is a great idea to print of a sheet that gives you the total carbs for each vegetable as a guide. If you want to follow what I did, for most days I ate the LOWEST carb veggies at dinner time. I could get away with eating 400-500g of bok choy with a little broccoli if I wanted each night (which filled my up alongside my meat) and still be for the whole day under 20g TOTAL carbs, which gets you loosing fat weight.

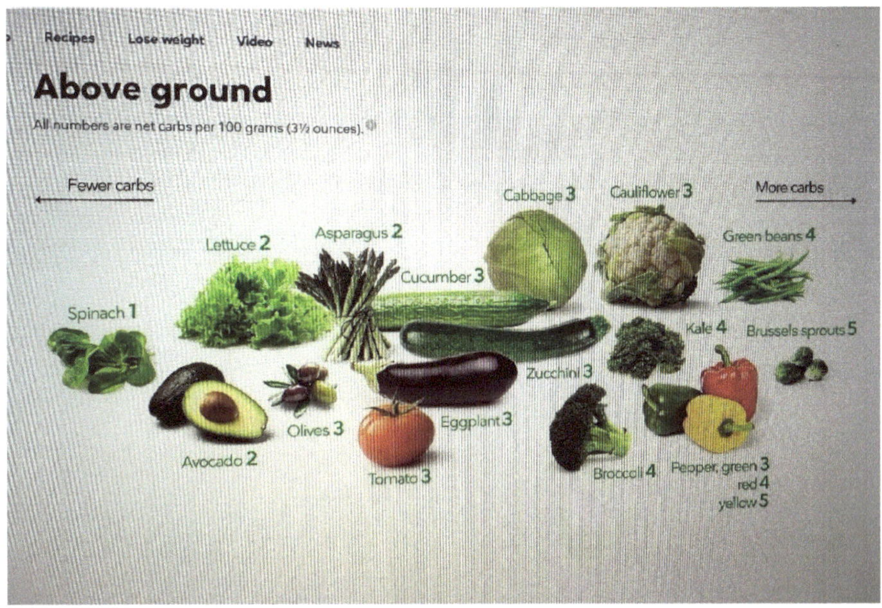

- All foods may be cooked in a microwave, oven, baked, boiled, stir fried, roasted, fried, grilled or sautéed. No flour, cornmeal, cornstarch or breading is allowed, that's empty high carbs!

FOODS YOU SHOUD EAT EVERYDAY, at least 2 cups:
Arugula
Bok choy
Cabbage (all versions)
Chard

Chives
Endive
Greens
Kale
Lettuce
Parsley
Spinach
Radicchio
Radishes
Scallions (spring onions)
Watercress

FIBROUS VEGETABLES include:
Asparagus
Broccoli
Brussel sprouts
Bamboo shoots
Bean sprouts Cauliflower
Celery (gorgeous with blue cheese crumbles and sour cream dip I make myself, simply mash a tablespoon of sour cream with the blue cheese with a fork and you'll have a potent amazing blue cheese dip!)

Celeriac (celery root)
Chayote
Cucumber
Edamame beans
Eggplant
Fennel
Green beans
Jicama
Mushrooms (be careful, higher in carbs)
Okra
Pepper
Pumpkin
Rhubarb
Rutabaga (swede)
Snow peas
Sprouts (bean and alfalfa)
Sugar snap peas
Summer squash
Tomatoes (but I had none from the start until now which today I 1st July 2018)
Turnip

Wax beans
Zucchini (courgetti)

BOULLION:
Have up to 2 cups for day one to day 4 or 5. This will help with your sodium replenishment as after day 2 or 3 of keto you can feel weak. This is a good sign, it signals that your body is stopping burning sugar for its energy source and its converting over to burning fat sources for its primary energy source. Your about to enter your body becoming a FAT BURNING MACHINE. All those excess fat stores will begin to be utilized by the body to fuel your brain and body functions, this is exactly what you want to start shedding those unwanted pounds one week at a time!

Drinking clear broth is strongly recommended. It will help avoid headaches and fatigue as your body adjusts to your new diet and switches over into becoming a fat burner, in other words when your body goes into a state call KETOSIS. What would be a great thing to do at the start as I did was buy Ketone testing strips at Walmart opposite the pharmacy, on the shelf. That is a test that will after 15 seconds tell you if you're in ketosis. When the body starts burning fat it releases ketones which are also detectable in small amounts in this diet in the urine. It served as a motivation tool for me coupled with the weekly phenomenal weight loss.

You can eat mayonnaise, up to 4 tablespoons a day. Dukes and Hellmann's are low carb. Always check the label of other brands, make sure the carb count is low on everything (under 2g) per serving.

FATTY VEGETABLES
Olives have up to 6 a day
Avocado have up to ½ of it a day.

CONDIMENTS:
Lemon/lime juice have up to 2 tablespoons a day.
Soy sauces have up to 4 tablespoons a day. Kikkoman is a low carb brand. Check the labels on other brands.
Mayonnaise

FATS AND OILS
Only real butter that has two ingredients, sweet cream and salt (if you like salted butter)
Coconut oil
Lard

Olive oil
Any other natural oil
Blue cheese, ranch, Caesar and Italian dressings (even store brought) are allowed if their carbohydrates say 1 or 2gs per serving or less.
You can add fat sources to salads like chopped eggs, bacon and or grated cheese.

Fats from natural sources (meats, eggs, avocados, oil, butter) are exceptional at making food taste good and do a good job of your stomach reaching that full satisfied feeling. This is also what decreases and makes sugar cravings go away completely too, coupled with filling your stomach up on veggies! I found from day one by eating these allowed foods I did not once crave a sugar fix or sweet carbohydrate fix like break or pasta. You will be ok, but it may be different for different people what your experience might be. overall you will transition on this lifestyle change and within the first week at some point. Let's be clear, you are not following a low-fat diet (that is not needed or not what this is about).

SNACKS:
You got to have snacks available. Reaching for the right one will keep you always on track. Dedicate a shelf for you at home with all the snacks and other condiments you can eat. It focuses you to you and keeps your head and mind on your lifestyle change.
Pork rinds
Pepperoni slices
Ham
Beef
Turkey
Other meat roll ups
Deviled eggs
Costco's seaweed squares, organic roasted seaweed. Carbs are next to nothing!
Parmesan chips (these have 0g carbs but watch the calories though, not too much in one day).

WHEN YOU ARE HUNGRY EAT YOUR CHOICE OF THE FOLLOWING: MEAT, POULTRY OR FISH/ SHELLFISH

MEAT:
Beef
Pork (bacon part of this obviously)
Lamb, veal or others

Processed meats like sausages, pepperoni, hot dogs (just read their carb content which should be about 1g per serving, anything more is too much)

POULTRY
Chicken
Turkey
Duck
Any other foul

FISH AND SHELLFISH
Tuna
Salmon
Catfish
Bass
Trout
Shrimp
Scallops
Crab
Lobster
(Please consider avoiding farmed seafood, there are too many toxins in them).

EGGS
Allowed without really any restriction but do add up your total carbohydrate count in the 'Loose it' app. You'll quickly see what amount you can get away with depending on what you eat for the day. I always had 2 to 3 meals a day and some days with snacks. Most of my early days ended up being a total of 15-20g TOTAL (not net) carbs for the day. This is what truly helped me see the weekly weight loss amounts shared with you in chapter 7.

SWEETNERS
If you feel the need to eat or drink something sweet (I never did as my taste changed and once the sugar was out of my body I never craved anything sweet. I never did want or need something sweet from March 26th, 2018 until currently 1st July 2018 and I have gone from 180.1 lbs. to 144 lbs. to date 1st July 2018. These are exact true figures and the scale and compliments I get from people, don't lie!)

Splenda (sucralose)
Nutra- sweet (aspartame)
Truvia (stevia/ erythritol blend
Pure organic stevia

Sweet n low (saccharin)

BEVERAGES
Water, from day one I got a 1-liter cup from Walmart and added my own straw. It had to be one liter (it was hard to find) because I made up my mind to drink at least 4 cup full's per day so I could congratulate myself on drinking a gallon a day. I would mark each cup drank down as a tally on my calendar, so I knew where I was at.

The best beverage is water.

Fizzy sugar free cans/ drinks as well as sparkling water are good choices.

Clear broth/ bullion (not low sodium, no added sugar)

CAFFEINATED BEVERAGES
You can have ONE of the following per day like I did
1.   3 cups of coffee (with or without heavy whipping cream and artificial sweetener)
2.   6 cups of tea
3.   3 caffeinated diet sodas
Or mix and match slightly.

CREAM
Sour cream, up to 4 tablespoons a day
Heavy whipping cream, light whipping cream (not half and half)

CHEESE
Hard
Swiss
Cheddar (my absolute favorite which I used only to flavor my spring mix salads for lunch, it was my staple lunch 126g spring mix salad from BJ's and 40g sharp cheddar cheese cut into tiny pieces and dispersed through salad. This lunch is only 5g total carbs. No dressing did I need, and it was DELICIOUS! I repeated this lunch over and over because it was quick and easy to prepare and take with me. It kept me to until dinner with drinking water in-between or green/ peppermint tea without sweetener).

Brie
Camembert
Blue cheese
Mozzarella (yes you can have a type of pizza with this cheese and pepperoni baked on parchment paper under the broiler and add some diced jalapenos

or put mozzarella inside a cut jalapeno and place some pepperoni slices on top and grill in broiler. It satisfied a pizza craving for me!

Gruyere
Cream cheese
Goat chesses
Feta
Parmesan

Always as with everything, check the label and make sure the carbohydrate count is less than 1 g per serving with chesses.

DESSERTS
Unsweetened shredded coconut flakes
Canned coconut milk (organic Wholefoods 365 brand is excellent)
Lindt 90% dark chocolate (if your macros allow it roughly then have 4 squares and you can have that every night and still succeed in loosing weight, even though it contains sugar. This has been done by a lady I know who lost 170 lbs. on keto which did take her 2 years and every night she had 4 squares of 90% cacao dark chocolate by Lindt!)

WHAT YOU CAN EAT EATING OUT GUIDE
If you're eating out (can be a significant part of most people's lives) do not be afraid or feel guilty about asking for a meal minus the bun or a slightly different order to what's listed in the menu. You're paying good money for it, they will accommodate you and know that you do not need to explain yourself either.

YOU CAN EAT
INDIAN
Almost anything but avoid rice, lentils, dahl.
Korma, eat as a thick soup (and no potatoes-based veggie dishes)

CHINESE
Pork spare ribs with no sauce
Roasted duck
Egg drop soup
Suan la tang
Hot and sour soup
Unbreaded prawns
Plain or unbattered wings

BURGER JOINTS
Any burger without the bun and sauces like ketchup
Salads instead of fries (most can offer salad alternatives instead of fries with a meal)

ITALIAN
Any oily salad with meatballs or cheese as a base (do ask if not on menu)
Italian sausage with different peppers
Any meat with marsala sauce, mostly veal or chicken
Pizza, just peel of the crust
Steaks and lobster
Acqua pazza
Omelets

JAPANESE
Sashimi
Teriyaki (beware of sweet sauces)

GOLDEN CORRAL (the only place I ate at during my weight loss period and maybe I only ate there 4 times)
Steak
Mushrooms
Salad with or without allowed dressings
Green cooked peppers with sautéed onion mix
Broccoli
Cauliflower
Buffalo wings
Sothern chicken just peel of breading coating
This is all I stuck to, and yes, it was never hard for me to watch my children and husband have all the dessert they wanted as I knew my focus and was filled to the brim with mainly steak!

CAFES AND BREAKFAST BARS
All day breakfasts are fine (bacon, eggs, sausage, minus the toast, scones, biscuits and waffles, obviously!)

MEXICAN
Chicken or steak fajita mix WITHOUT the tortillas, served on a bed of lettuce and sour cream with guacamole
Chipotle salads
Taco salad in general fine minus the shells (soft and hard)

Doing keto? Keep it simple stupid and lose weight with no exercise!

STEAKHOUSES
Steaks
Ribs without sauces
Burgers without buns
Salads with oily dressings or mayonnaise which is always allowed.

SEAFOOD RESTURANTS
All seafood good without the breading/batter/ sweet sauces
Mussels ONLY in moderation (higher in carbs, beware)

TURKISH
Kebab/gyro; get the meat on salad, skip the hummus. Dressing option that's best is mayo which is the lowest carb count.

VIETNAMESE
Pho without the noodles. Still has a little sugar but its worth it. Ask for extra sprouts.

GERMAN
Any meat without too much sugar potentials
Roasted plain meats
Steak Tartar
Sauerkraut

I will list my dessert that I love in chapter 10 and I did not need any dessert for most of the time during my short weight loss period naturally. I was content after that last dinner meal each day until sleeping.

3 WHAT FOODS YOU CAN'T EAT

Keto is a LOW CARB but moderate fat and protein diet. This is how I've been using it. All my carbs come from vegetables mainly and a little from my dessert which I list in chapter 10.
NO simple carbohydrates which no sugars are (hence no fruit initially) and no starches (these are complex carbohydrates and are not allowed as the body can break them down into sugars). The only carbohydrates encouraged are the nutritionally dense, fiber rich vegetables listed before.

YOU CAN'T EAT SUGARS (avoid anything containing):
White sugar
Brown sugar
Honey
Maple syrup
Molasses
Corn syrup
Beer (contains barley malt)
Milk whole or skimmed (contains a type of sugar called lactose)
Diary substitutes
Flavored yoghurts
Fruit juice
Fruit
Canned soups
Ketchup (unless its sugar free like Walden Farms brand)
Barbeque sauce (unless its sugar free like above, find on Vitacost)
Sweet condiments and relished
Half and half
Coffee creamer
Lite salad dressings (read their carbohydrate content, usually higher than 2g

per serving)
Avoid processed cheese such as Velveeta

YOU CAN'T EAT STARCHES (avoid the following kinds of foods):
Grains (yes, even whole grains)
Rice
Cereals
Flour
Cornstarch
Breads
Pastas
Muffins
Bagels
Crackers
Beans and legumes (pinto, lima, black beans, peas etc.)
Most root vegetables particularly carrots, parsnips, corn, potatoes, French fries, potato chips.

YOU CAN'T EAT SUGAR ALCOHOL SWEENTENERS
(Avoid foods with these sugar alcohols)
Sorbitol
Maltitol

MEATS: DO NOT EAT
Breading on meats (they are full of carbs)
Read the labels for carb count.

YOU CAN'T HAVE ALCOHOL INTITALLY
I got to my weight (March 26th, 2018 – July 1st, 2018 to 144 lbs.) without consuming any alcohol. Some ketogenic dieter does permit one glass of wine which you can do if your macros allow it (see if you have enough carbs left for the day to cover a glass on the Loose it app. A 50x glass of wine weighs out to 150g on a kitchen grams scale. This comes out to approximately 125 calories and about 4g of carbs. So, if your daily macro's and calories allow it you can go for it. The aim is to stay right around 20g od TOTAL carbs a day. I did not go by NET as NET allows more carbs in and I was serious about being on the quickest route to fat burning. I figured I could switch to net carb counting once reaching my goal to MAINTAIN my weight and not to go on loosing more.

4 KEEP IT SIMPLE STUPID & SUCCEED, MEAL PLAN!

You must keep things simple each week to succeed. This means deciding what it is you want for that 7 days for each meal, for breakfast, for lunch and for dinner. How I did it was shop for a week, once a week and I would write down my weekly shopping list after I had written down what I wanted my meals to be. This next thing is the most crucial step that helped me get through. I would tend to eat the SAME thing ALL WEEK. So yes, the same breakfast, lunch and dinner. It's not boring, it was still very enjoyable because I loved the food I was eating, and it was SIMPLE. I did not waste money or produce as I used it all up for the week. I could and did cook sometimes in that same week DIFFERENT things for my family (six children and my husband) but the simple fact of knowing precisely what I was having all week helped me massively.

I could then cook just chicken breast all week for dinner (have it marinating in the fridge in one go and take out each day and cook the rough amount needed) and be calm. It allowed me to prep and zip lock bag up my bok choy, kale and broccoli for the 6- 7 days ahead to sautéed to go with my dinner.

My lunches were the same for example, a $3 organic spring mix salad box from BJ's would last me about 4 days (which is just about its length of shelf life anyway) and I would eat that with 40g of sharp aged cheddar cheese and be excited to have that same dish each day that week as it tasted fabulous!

Breakfast would also be the same, whatever I had decided before writing my shopping list. Folks this is how I recommend you do this. I would like to have some weeks (all week long) one tin of sardines in olive oil with 40g spinach for breakfast or another week I would happily have eggs (fried in 14g of butter, (a knob) with a few strips of bacon. Meal planning is key, then from there you create your shopping list, then from there you only buy for that week what you will eat.

Don't forget to decide what your snacks will be. I love about 20g of pork rinds or roasted seaweed for mine. I did very well doing this, if I needed a snack.

I will warn you, eating this way, because my body had lots of fat stores, you will experience this… you will become LESS hungry. I had to drop a meal to two meals a day because of this as you MUS ONLY EAT WHEN YOUR HUNGRY. Why, you must do this to listen to your body. Your body will be in fat burning mode so when you start to experience no huger and realize that you can go longer without eating in-between meals THAT NORMAL and there's nothing wrong with you. It's because your body is utilizing your own body fat AS ITS FUEL! Your body is not running of the old fuel, the sugar/ carbohydrate fuel it had been probably all your life, it's now breaking down fat stores slowly but surely as you are not giving it glucose to burn. The body is forced to burn fat for energy.

Fat as a fuel is MORE efficient for the brain, so your mind will be sharper, and you should experience that you become better at doing your daily tasks, whilst being happy and content with all the good yummy food your allowed to eat!

Meal plan, then write your shopping list according to what your decided meals are. Even run your meal plan through the loose it app to theoretically see what your total macros would be should you consume that breakfast, lunch and dinner you choose. Play with quantities, see what your carbs total as and weigh on your kitchen scales accordingly. You'll soon become an expect at your own simple, uncomplicated choices.

Below are a couple of examples of what I exactly ate for the week and I am always exact as I measure my food and then plug the information into the loose it app, so I can share what my TOTAL carbs were for the day (which I would repeat all week long). Remember, go by TOTAL carbs.

WEEK ONE

Breakfast:

FOOD	TOTAL CARBS	NET CARBS	FIBRE
Spinach 40g Canned sardines in olive oil 124g	1.5g	0.6g	0.9g

Lunch:

FOOD	TOTAL CARBS	NET CARBS	FIBRE
2 eggs, 19g butter Seaweed 5g	0.3g	0.3g	0g

Dinner:

FOOD	TOTAL CARBS	NET CARBS	FIBRE
300g beef steak, 194g broccoli, 50g mushrooms	7.6g	1.1g	6.5g

So, see how easy it is to stay at 20g TOTAL carbs or less per day. Total carbs for this day was 9.4g. This was particularly low, but I was filled and needed to eat nothing more. Now because you can go up to 20g of total carbs you can now afford a dessert, or a glass of wine weighed out on a gram scale to 150g which will add for the wine alone another 3.9g of total carbs.

Doing keto? Keep it simple stupid and lose weight with no exercise!

Another week example… same all week

Breakfast:

FOOD	TOTAL CARBS	NET CARBS	FIBRE
Cheddar cheese 30g, 2 eggs Butter 5g	0.4g	0.4g	0g

Lunch:

FOOD	TOTAL CARBS	NET CARBS	FIBRE
Kimchee 113g	2g	1g	1g

Dinner:

FOOD	TOTAL CARBS	NET CARBS	FIBRE
Chicken breast pan fried 312g, Broccoli 150g, Bok choy 200g	8.9g	2.3g	6.6g

Total carbs for this day was 11.3g. If you know what your carbs are for each day you can rest assured that you will lose weight coupled with not exceeding your calorie budget for the day as given to you by the loose it app. That's how I did it. Most weeks, except a couple here and there, I did not go over the app's calorie budget it set for me. When you sign up it will figure an estimate to lose weight for your data you provide it. It's a truly great app, I LOVE it!

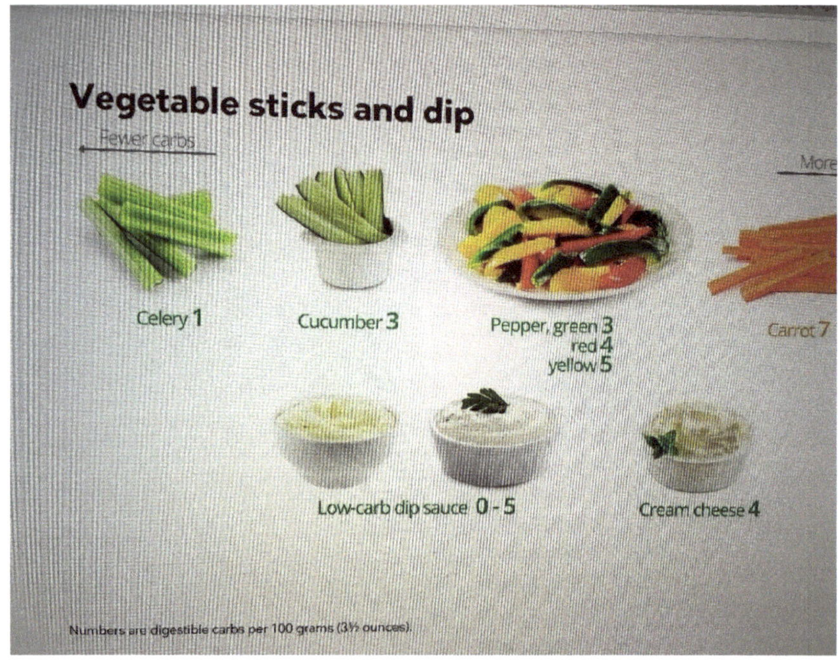

5 WHAT CARB RULE DID I FOLLOW

As you have probably gathered by now, I followed sticking to the prescribed drug version, the most potent version for the quickest and most effective weight loss, the TOTAL CARB counting. Stayed at or below 20 g of carbohydrate eaten per day!

Follow this and you will lose weight and I dare to say you will even lose weight if you go a bit over your calories consumption as the carbohydrate count is what is kept.

Without carbs your body is forced to look for another source of fuel, that's energy to breath, and do all the wonderful things it does. It must get it from fat. Now this can be fat on your body and or fat that you eat. For the beginning you can even go a step further in accelerating your body being a fat burning machine FROM YOUR OWN stores, that is to opt for more leaner meats. Less fat on meats will equal more fat burning for energy from your own body fat. However, eating fat will always still allow you to lose your body fat, maybe not as fast.

6 WHT SYMPTOMS TO EXPECT THE FIRST THREE DAYS OF STARTING KETO

Well you will hear on you tube people calling these symptoms the 'keto flu'. The symptoms I only experience was on the morning of the second day was not so nice weakness, after I had awoken from my bed and stood up, I was feeling weak inside all over really. I had to slowly get ready and then once I was dressed I went to the kitchen and I had to sit down, something I never normally ever have to do. I remember it like yesterday.

It was not dizziness, just weakness. This was a sign that all my sugar (glucose) in my body was used up and my body momentarily did not have fuel to provide energy until it had switched itself over to breaking down fat stores and or utilizing some fat from what I had eaten for its primary energy source, importantly to fuel the brain. Our brains and muscles need a constant supply of energy and until that transition fully clicked over I was left feeling weak to the point I had to sit. I remember thinking I must get up and make my children's breakfast. I got up and got my water and sat down with it straight away and drank a liter. Within minutes my weakness went away, I was so pleased that water alone fixed me so quickly. I then proceeded with my tasks.

Note at the point I reached to drink water, you can avoid most of any symptoms involved with transitioning from your body being a sugar burner to a fat burner by drinking either bullion (chicken or beef) with salt from day one. You may therefore never experience any symptoms as it will replenish your water/ electrolyte and chemical balance. There is a lot of water weight loss in that first week too so drinking a gallon a day will help with everything. As you will see in the chapter 7, even though I drank a gallon of water each day AND ate my food, my weight loss was massive! So, shall yours be.

This will spur you on and give you the all needed incentive to keep at it. Because this keto lifestyle change is enjoyable and you're not hungry, you'll find it easy to make it a way of life and you will never go back overall. You'll enjoy see the weight loss like I did.

7 MY WEEKLY WEIGHT LOSS RESULTS

My weight recording happens EVERY Tuesday morning as soon as I wake up, and to get a true recording consistently each time I do so after the first restroom visit upon arising out of bed and void of clothes. Below are the dates and the weight I was on those wonderful Tuesday's.

I always look forward to weighing myself now on this lifestyle and I will always do it to see if I'm doing well at maintain my desired weight where I am now. No more can those horrid pounds creep up on me as I will act against it by lowering my carbs in my diet and the best part I've been relieved about, I did this weight loss with only two sessions on the treadmill for 20 minutes each. Exercise is NOT needed to get these results!

DATE (Tuesday's)	WEIGHT RECORDED IN LBS
March 27th 2018	180.1
April 3rd 2018	170.9
April 10th 2018	166.3
April 17th 2018	166.3 stayed the same, does happen
April 24th 2018	163.8
May 1st 2018	162.0
May 8th 2018	160.5
May 15th 2018	160.5 stayed the same, be patient
May 22nd 2018	156.5
May 29th 2018	158.2 I over ate at golden corral
June 5th 2018	155.8
June 12th 2018	151.7

June 19th 2018	155.3 over ate golden corral night before
June 26th 2018	144.5 much more water drinking .

Here I currently am, I'm at 144.5. My goal for my height was 150 lbs. I've exceeded that and now all I must do is MAINTAIN it. You saw how a little over indulgence on steak can put a couple of pounds on in one week so be careful. But providing you don't go too crazy and introduce over 30g of total carbs a day you will easily the next week shed that gained weight as the body will burn it off, but you must stay true to keto. Otherwise you will go out of ketosis and it usually takes about 3 to 5 days to get back in.

overall, I stayed and still stay in a ketosis state, I.e. my body is a fat burning machine and I love that! People who you no doubt will get to listen too on you tube will tell how they successfully maintained their desired weight after losing it this way for 7 plus years so that's amazing. I can honestly say that I will be having no troubles in doing the same. Go keto!!

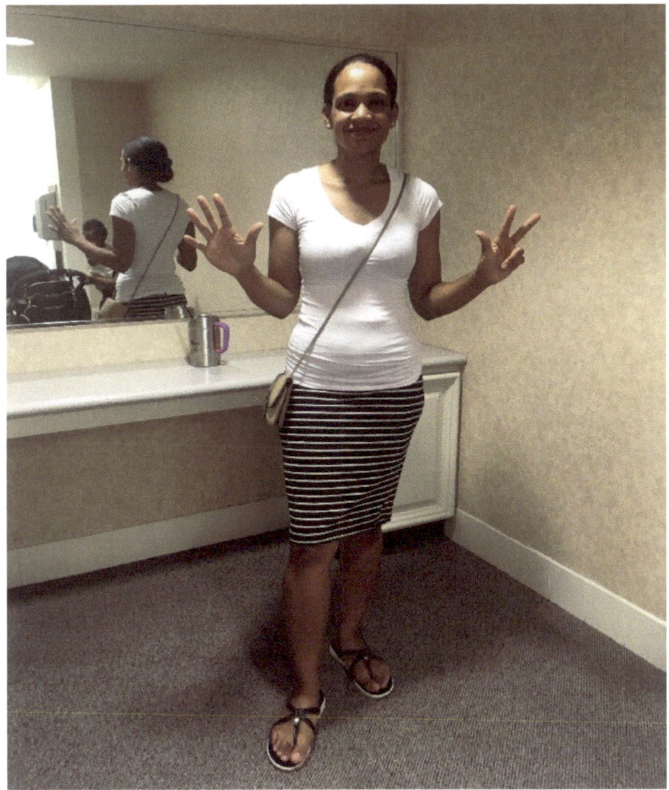

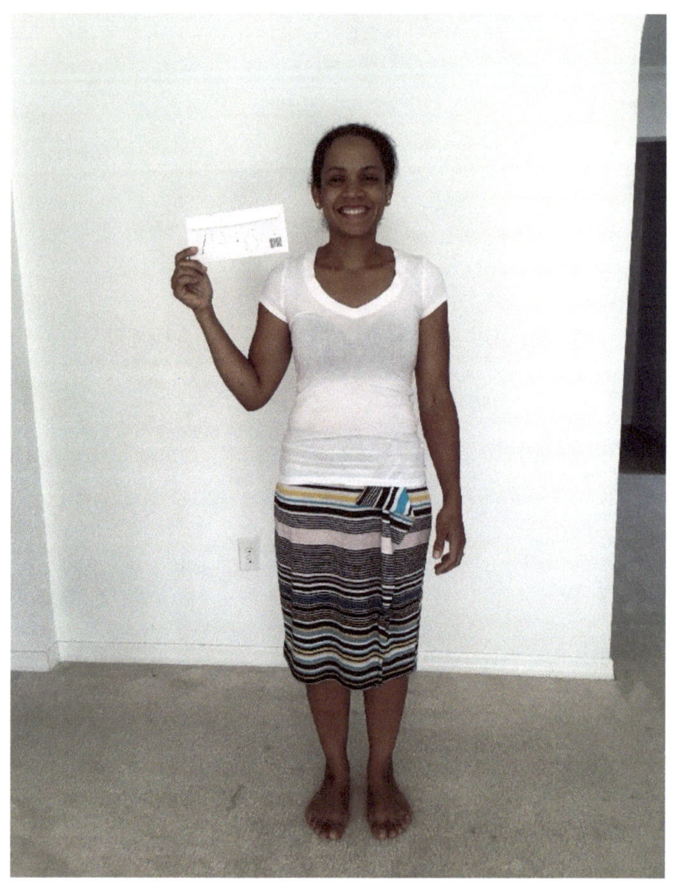

8 MEASURING TOOLS AND KEEPING FOCUSED

What I had were a kitchen scale, to measure my foods including butter I used to fry eggs, fish and sauté my veg. This was so I could count my carbs by plugging in the data int the 'loose it' app.

I also from day one brought keto strips from Walmart, they can be found somewhere near the pharmacy counter and are around 46 to buy. You do not need a prescription to get them, just pick them off the counter like you would toothpaste. They are test strips to test the ketone level in your urine and ketone levels are normally highest on day two of starting keto, showing a moderate level. They are always higher in the evenings throughout your life being keto.

I have had a good number of mornings where I tested my ketone levels with a negative result on these strips. I did worry a little that I was out of ketosis but when you look at my steady weight loss, I clearly was in a good state all along, it's just that experts and doctors say that ketone levels are lower in the mornings compared to the evenings. Also, you need to understand that as the body starts using ketones (which are the byproduct of fat breaking down) for fuel it gets more and more efficient at taking them up and using them for fuel, so the number of ketones present in the urine will go down that way, because the body is successfully using more of those ketones for fuel.

I also used a body weighing scale, weighing once a week on Tuesdays. This was the greatest form of encouragement. In the first week I reported an almost 10 lbs. weight loss. They say out there that this is mostly water but still, I've never in my entire life lost 10 lbs. on any kind of diet before in 7 days, so if you only have 10 lbs. to lose, fortunate you! You'll be at your goal in 7 days!

I also used a measuring tape. I measured my hips and smallest part of my waist twice in this short time frame.

Here are my results which I recorded in my personal email.

When I weighed 180.1 lbs. at the beginning my waist measured in at 32.5 inches and my hips at 41 inches.

It's quite incredible to know the facts of measurements because now I can see in addition to the weight on the scale, what proportions my body was changing to.

My next set of measurement I took on 1st June 2018 and my waist were 29 inches and my hips were 33inches. To me that's amazing.

Everywhere I go now, to all my regular shops, people are complimenting my weight loss as I had weight 200 lbs. after giving birth to my now 15-month-old baby and had stayed around 185 lbs. for 15 months. So, everyone knew I was bigger for all that time until suddenly starting this way of life on keto, it took me 3 months, 12 weeks to be at my ideal goal weight and I lost a total of 35.6 lbs. with hardly any exercise, just doing what I did running around after six children as I did before when I was at 180.1 lbs.

It was not me being active with the children that got me where I am today but the application of adopting a keto based lifestyle did it, through food choices. You can achieve the same results in such little time if you want to.

Be inspired! I truly wish you all the success and wisdom that comes from this ketogenic way of life.

9 MY WEIRD EXPERIENCE OF NOT FEELING HUNGRY

Doctors who have treated their diabetic patients to get them off insulin have reported that their patients will natural reduce the appetite by eating a low carb diet such as this ketogenic one. The hunger disappears for longer periods of time. When that starts to happen please listen to it and only eat when hungry.

We have become so accustomed to eating three to five meals a day by habit, but this has probably been maintained by the level of carbohydrate intake we've always done without much thought. It has been my experience about four weeks into this way of eating that I noticed that I was simply NOT hungry at breakfast time and I wouldn't eat until 1 or 2pm. It was only by 1-2pm that I began to start feeling hungry, so I just listened and obeyed to only eat when I started to feel hungry. I did have a little thought at the time saying, 'what's wrong with me, why aren't I hungry'. When I researched about it, I quickly learnt that I was not the only one and that was normal.

What the body was doing is that it was steadily getting its required source of energy from your internal fat stores, breaking it down and fueling itself so it had no need to signal to you that it was hungry.

What's fascinating is that the body cannot even access its own fat stores if you eat any kind of sugar or over eat on carbohydrates (which the body breaks down into sugar very very easily) because of the insulin rise in the blood. Eating sugar raises the blood insulin almost immediately and when that insulin is raised, energy is burnt from sugar and not from fat stores and if you don't burn all that sugar insulin tells the body to lock it away as fat eventually, first as glycogen, which is a sugar store in the liver and then to adipose tissue which is the medical term for fat tissue. The aim of the game is to keep insulin at the lowest possible level for most of the time which unlocks your body's ability to go in and use those fat stores you don't want to carry around! Dr Fung teaches bout this in connection to intermittent fasting and it's all so fascinating. When you finally get to understand the mechanism of how our marvelous bodies work you will feel a sense of empowerment with that knowledge.

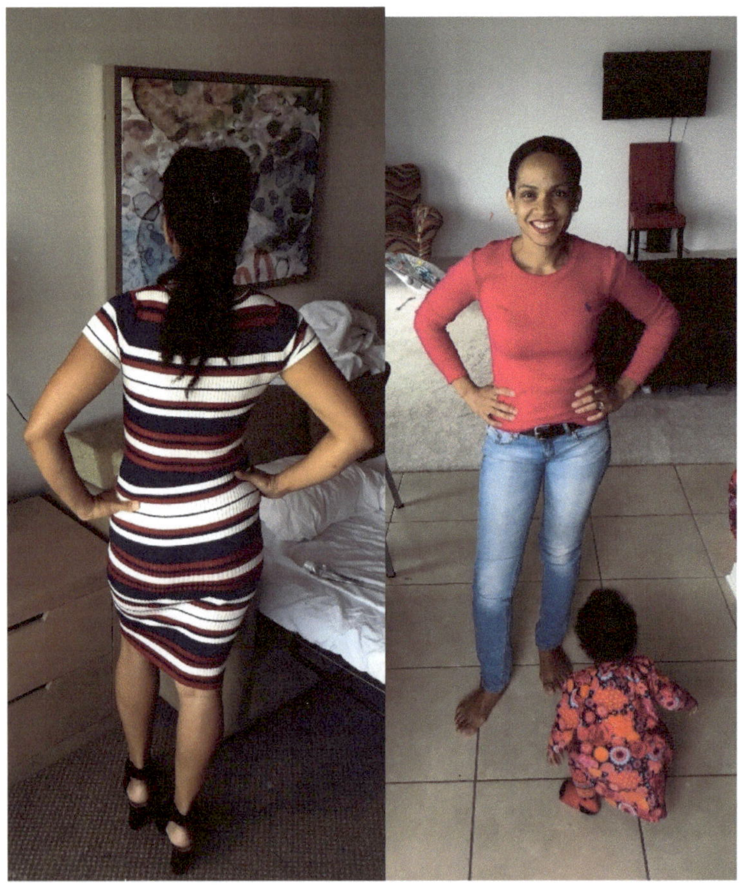

10 MY 10 TOP MEALS AND DESSERT PLUS MY 7 KETO TIPS

TEN TOP MEALS
1. 500g roasted chicken wings with skin on with 12 celery sticks, 10 tablespoons of Franks hot sauce, 2 tablespoons of sour cream with 60g of blue cheese mashed in the sour cream
2. 417g pan fried salmon in 18g butter, 100g sautéed kale and 45g green bell pepper
3. 312g chicken breast, 150g broccoli sautéed in same pan after chicken was cooked
4. Steak 220g, chicken liver pans fried 200g, 500g bok choy, 19g crumbled goats cheese
5. 350g top round eye steak, 500g bok choy, 19g butter for sautéing veg. (Whatever roast I do I would roast it all at the start of the week and carve it up per day and weigh it out, making life simple and easier).
6. 400g Jamaican curry goat (I buy from Golden Krust take away or sometimes cook my own), 150g broccoli, 20g mushrooms.
7. 450g prawns with tail on, sautéed in real garlic and 15g butter, squeeze of lemon juice in the mix and salt and pepper. Served with 200g sautéed diced okra.
8. 450g oxtail in bone broth and 500g bok choy
9. Cauliflower rice cooked with garlic, salt and pepper served with 400g pan fried salmon on top
10. 350g Beef eye of round roast with 200g spring salad and a mixture of feta and goats cheese crumbles on top, with side of sauerkraut

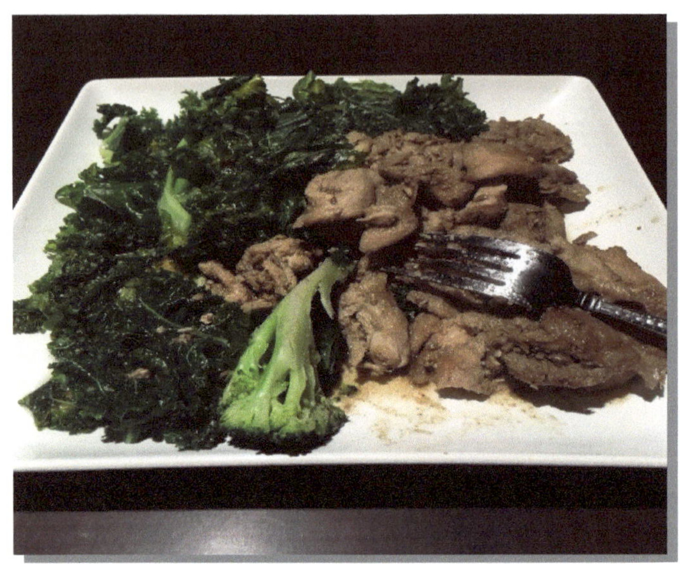

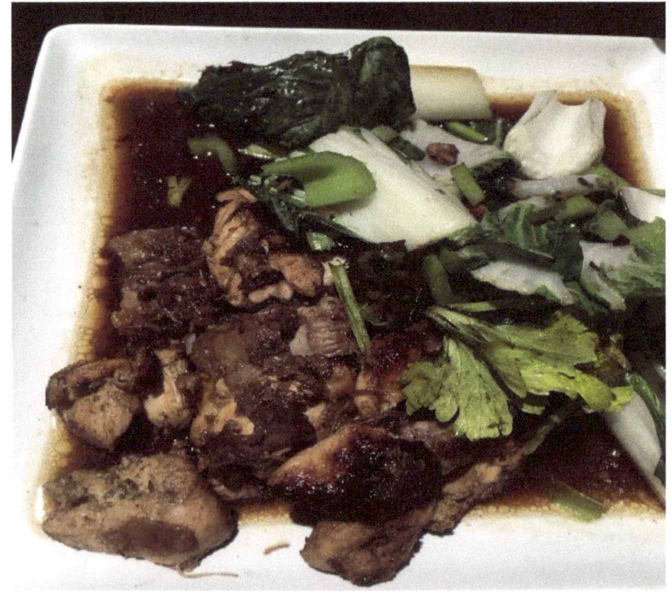

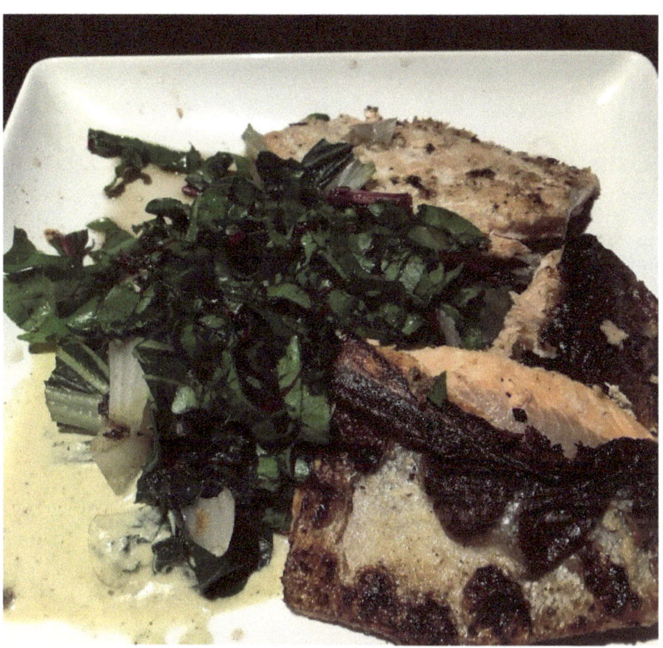

MY TWO DESSERTS

1. Creamy dreamy coconut dessert: only two ingredients, 80 mls of wholefoods organic 365 canned coconut milk with 14g of organic unsweetened shredded coconut flakes. Mix together and eat.

This dessert was immediately sweet enough for me. My palate could taste the natural sweetness in here but if you need anything sweeter I recommend reaching for organic stevia. Also, this is a pleasure to eat as it takes about 10 mins to eat so savor it. The time is prolonged because of chewing that lovely coconut shreds. Normally desserts can be gone in five minutes or less. I self-discovered this dessert and fell in love with it after I had a surplus of shredded coconut in my pantry!

2. Cream cheesecake fluff: 2 oz of Philadelphia or Walmart's great value brand of soft cream cheese and stevia to sweeten slightly. mix, eat and enjoy!

MY 7 KETO TIPS

1. If your serious about loosing your excess fat faster, eat meat and vegetables not fat from all different fat sources too much. This will further encourage your body to burn the fat from your body instead. Lots of ketogenic dieters say keto is low carb and high fat, moderate to high protein but if you're looking to lose weight don't

provide your body with high fat.

2. Focus on eating real whole foods. You don't have to buy special ingredients or supplements if you want to keep keto simple. Focus on the OUTER perimeter of the grocery store, where the meats, the cheeses, the eggs and the diary-based products are like sour cream, whipping creams are.

3. When first starting keto, if your used to eating 3 meals a day then stick to that and replace those meals with the foods you can eat or cut out the foods you can't eat. Don't start out with any kind of intermittent fasting either, I've only introduced that at three months in for the health rewards, of which you can research about. You can do 'lazy keto' which is where you don't measure out anything but still eat ketogenic friendly foods and you will still loose the weight as you cut out all breads, pasta, wheat, cakes, biscuits etc. You are bound to lose weight just by doing this. If your used to eating breakfast switch cereal for eggs and bacon.

4. Tip to keep keto simple, MEAL PLAN. Do a once a week shopping trip and write down what your going to buy, keeping it simple stupid! You will end up eating everything you buy for that week, keeping the meals the same for that week.

5. Drink a gallon or try to drink at least minimum 3 liters of water a day. It will regulate your body and flush you and most times curb hunger for a while. Sometimes when you feel a slight hunger about to start water drinking can make that stay away for over an hour or more.

6. Keto snacks are essential to have with you just in case you must eat something and will keep you on track of staying in ketosis with no setbacks.

7. Avoid snacking at bedtime, differentiate between head hunger and stomach hunger also. Go to bed at bedtime. How do you differentiate between head hunger and stomach hunger? Well stomach huger is that hunger you feel in your stomach, that achy empty feeling accompanied by some rumbling. You feel this when you haven't eaten in a while. That's different to head hunger. Head hunger is what I would describe as that feeling that you just want to eat but you don't know why or maybe you have a headache or feel unhappy or tiered and maybe you just want to feel good, or your bored and ant to feel entertained by eating something. That's what I would describe as head hunger and not to action that type. Either find something else to do or just go to bed and sleep. It will be much better for you.

ABOUT THE AUTHOR

I am 37 years old and began this ketogenic way of eating at this age. Before discovering it, I was feeling down that my weight was remaining the same despite cutting back on unhealthy snacks and cakes. Little did I know that the amount of natural sweeteners like honey and maple syrup as well as eating no end of raisins, fruits like bananas, apples and grapes were keeping me at my undesired weight, I was very fortunate to discovered and out into practice what I had learnt from research. I still happily take care of all my children while my husband works, and I am so so thrilled that my weight has ticked down and down on the scale all because I've changed my food choices to keto friendly ones.

I embrace all my (new) clothes as I went from 180.1 lbs. to 144.5 lbs. in 3 months, losing a total of 35.6 lbs. effortlessly, except the effort to meal plan! It's so rewarding to get out of size 12 clothes and fit into a size 4! I can't begin to tell you how that feels. I can't really get over how quick it took. The compliments you will receive will tell you that you aren't going back to all that excess weight. You'll be the one to make sure of that, trust me. That's where I am now.